"Angels in the Valley------Poems, Prayers, Promises and helpful information for those with cancer and their caregivers"

By

Patti Sassy Angel Chiappa

1

Ordering Information:

Quantity sales. Special discounts are available on quantity purchases by corporations, associations, and others. For details, contact the publisher at the address above.

Orders by U.S. trade bookstores and wholesalers. Contact: Soulbabylondon@gmail.com

Printed in the United States of America 2016

This book is dedicated to all the angels who have a heart filled with faith even though they are going through their own valley. For all their wonderful care givers who encourage, love and give. For my dear family and friends who have lost their battle with cancer. My great aunt Viola, Uncle Walter, Uncle Willie, Aunt Mary Chiappa Uncle Al, Uncle Joe, Diana, Kyle, Sherry, Grandpa Fred, my beloved father Bernie, Aunt Dot, Great grandma, Aunt Roberta, Jane Hood, Diane Chiodo, Belinda Spatuntna, Mrs. Richard, Mr. Butler. For those who are still battling cancer, my friend Janice Sweet. Your courage, strength and light will always be a part of me.

Thank you for being a true inspiration. For the ones that encouraged me to write this book after my own" Tumor" scare, thank you for your support and listening ears. This book is for all of you. May the scriptures, poems and prayers bring you comfort and peace? A portion of this book profits will be donated to the Dana Farber Fund. Together we can kick cancer's ass!

Chapter One

"But your dead will live. Their bodies will rise. You who dwell in the dust wake up and shout for joy. Your dew is like the dew of morning. The earth will give birth to her dead."- Isaiah 26:19

The first time I ever heard the word "Cancer." I was only four years old. I did not know what the word meant, but I knew there was a lot of pain associated with it. It was my fourth birthday. My family had gathered around me to watch me blow out my candle on my birthday cake. My great aunt Viola with her gentle blue eyes and soft smile began to cry." I have breast cancer." She announced.

I recall looking around the room at my family members. The ones who were just smiling were now angry, lost and full of disbelief.

I recall turning to my great aunt. A woman that was so spiritual, so beautiful, so gentle, a woman I thought was an actual angel and said," What is cancer? "My great aunt the woman who taught me about prayer and faith and forgiveness took me by my little hand and replied," Cancer, is a way God brings us closer to him. It is a way that God teaches us to rely on our faith. It is a way that God shows us how strong we are.

Cancer, darling is an illness that makes people sick but it also makes them cherish every moment, every sunrise, every sunset, every song they hear, every smile they see, every hug they give and receive, every kiss and every day."

I looked at my aunt and asked," Are you going to die?" My aunt replied," I may leave this earth but I will be starting my new life with Jesus in Heaven."

"When Jesus entered the ruler's home and he saw the flute players and the noisy crowd he said," Go away! The girl is not dead but asleep. But they laughed at him. After the crowd had been put outside, he went and took the girl by the hand and she got up." Matthew 9:23 TO 9:25

After my fourth birthday, my great aunt ended up in the hospital. She began receiving chemo treatments. She had lost weight. She her lost her hair and energy but not her loving spirit. Whenever I saw her, she would do something to make me laugh. Her body had changed but not her beautiful smile, loving personally or gentle heart.

I saw how my family overcame the beast called Cancer through faith, prayer and togetherness. Even at an early age I began to understand that cancer can never rob memories, a person's spirit, the love of family and friends but most of all a person's faith. I understood that Jesus would stand by a person through good and bad, rain or sunshine, faith or fear.

The most important thing I learned from my aunt was that the same God on the mountain was the same God in the valley below. I saw God through my aunt's eyes. I saw that at her most desperate time of need that when she was reaching out to God, he was reaching back. "God will never leave you." She said to me the last time I saw her. "No matter what happens. God Will never leave you."

The night before my aunt died, I had a beautiful dream. I was engulfed by peace and comfort when I saw my beautiful aunt happy and healthy walking arm and arm with Jesus. My aunt was wearing a long and flowing white dress. Her hair was very thick and hung in little curls. My aunt smiled at me saying," By his stripes I am healed." She then kissed me on the head.

I said," Bye Auntie." The next night my grandma and my godfather watched Aunt Viola took her last breath.

The day we buried Aunt Viola it was a beautiful spring day. New buds bloomed on the trees, perfume from roses peppered the air, and a bring yellow sun warmed our faces. I was seven. For three years my family had been ironically been bonded by cancer. We had learned to make every day count, how to sacrifice but most inporantally how to pray as a family.

It was April 23, 1981 when we said our final goodbyes to a woman who inspired us to live every day to the fullest. It was aunt's battle with cancer that taught me the meaning of this scripture. From Luke 12: 8, "I tell you, whoever publicly acknowledges me before others, the Son of Man will also acknowledge before the angels of

God." On April 23, 1981 I did not weep for my aunt for I knew that she had left this earth to start her new life with Jesus. My aunt Viola had never given up on prayer. She never became bitter or angry. She never blamed God for her illness. She actually thanked God for allowing her to learn through her battle that she was strong, to enjoy every moment with your family and to love those around you.

Chapter 2

"Whatever happens abide steadfast in determination to simply cling to God." St. Francis De Sales.

My grandfather Fred was my hero. As a young man he worked selling pretzels in Madison Square Garden for just pennies a day. He was a stern German with a fighting spirit. He was a care giver, a male nurse during the War. A husband that would sacrifice anything for his wife. A father who was devoted. A grandfather full of wonderful advice. A friend to all. He was also the second person close to me that was stricken with cancer.

My grandfather was diagnosed with stomach cancer in the late 1980s. When he was diagnosed we just would not accept it. My grandfather was the patriarch of our family. He was strong and brave. He was a man that was bigger than life himself with his hardy laugh and booming voice. He was a warrior.

It was because my grandpa was this strong manly man that our family could not accept that cancer claimed his cells. We together as a family declared war against my grandfather's cancer.

We changed my grandpa's diet, tried alternative medicines, prayed and gave my grandpa's cancer over to God. We just would not let cancer claim him. Grandpa was just as determined to stay with us as we were of keeping him here. He was too stubborn to let cancer take him away from his family. Grandpa spent his days hiding his pain from us so we would not fear. We spent our days giving grandpa a reason to stay here.

"Strength is born in the deep silence of long suffering hearts not amidst joy." Felicia Hermans.

It was a cold Thanksgiving day when my grandfather had part of his colon removed. The doctor's warn us he may not survive the surgery. But we laughed in the face of their warning. They did not know how big our God was or how tough grandpa was. The day came for my grandpa's surgery. The whole family and out pastor gathered at the Hospital. We spent seven hours praying as my grandfather went under the knife.

Almost eight hours passed when a tried and weary surgeon walked out of the O.R. with tears in his eyes saying," He made it. He made it." In a joyful voice.

When we saw my grandpa in the recovery room in a horse and groggy voice he said," I'm hungry!"

We knew at that moment that grandpa was going to be fine.

Our family celebrated Thanksgiving that year at a Long Island Hospital. We ate our Thanksgiving meal off plastic trays but it was our best Thanksgiving ever. My grandfather returned home after only three days amazing all the doctors and beating the odds!

It was one doctor in particular that was deeply touched by my grandfather's victory. A Jewish man, he had rejected the idea that Jesus existed in his life until he met my grandpa. So moved by the miracle he saw, the doctor questioned my grandfather about his flawless faith. My grandfather simple explained to the doctor that he knew Jesus existed because he saw him everywhere he looked. In the eyes of his loved ones, in the rain, in flowers, in the pail moonlight. My grandfather had then shared with the doctor his favorite scripture. Psalm 9:10 New International Version. "Those who know your name trust in you, for you, LORD, have never forsaken those who seek you."

So astonished by my grandfather's healing, the devout Jewish man gave his heart to Jesus in the presence of a man whom Jesus healed from stage four cancer! Later on this man, this doctor brought his family to the heart of

Christ as well. My grandfather went on to have many happy and joyful years with our family.

Grandma and Grandpa got to celebrate their 50 wedding anniversary by renewing their vows in a beautiful and romantic ceremony. I will never forget it for a s long as I live. It was Feb 4, 1991. It was a snowy afternoon. My family went to 5 O'clock mass with my grandparents. At a church my grandparents had attended for 40 years. My grandfather was an usher and elder at the church. He had planned the entire event without any of us knowing about it. He had told my mom, dad, brother and I to get really dressed up because we were going to go out to dinner after church. So we did.

My brother and I were very excited because we loved going to dinner with my grandparents. During the mass I noticed my grandfather was smiling from ear to ear.

After church was over, my grandfather sprung the lovely surprise on all of us. The man who had survived brutal cancer got down on one knee and proposed to my grandma all over again.

My grandma, the little fireball who stood at only five feet tearfully accepted but then hit my grandfather playfully on the backside for not telling her what he was up too.

I got to be my grandma's maid of honor. My brother was my grandpa's best man. We tearfully, joyfully witnessed how a Christ centered marriage could endure the most testing trails, most pouring rains and shaky roads.

My heart swells with happiness as I recall how my grandfather called grandma his Florence Nightingale as he recited his vows. How after the breathtaking ceremony was over how he proudly told everyone at the church how God healed him and that my grandma's love was the core of his healing!

For years after my grandfather won his battle with cancer, he got to enjoy building wonderful memories, he got to see his grandchildren fall in love, dance many polkas with grandma and play many songs on his organ.

"Faith never knows where it is needed but it loves and knows the one who is leading." Oswald Chambers.

The second time my grandfather was diagnosed with cancer, this time kidney cancer we once again declared war!

This time my grandfather was much older and fragile then the last time. None of us believed however the God would simply decide that it was time for Grandpa to go home.

My grandfather's health declined very rapidly. It was a matter of weeks before he was bedridden and grandma became a full-time caretaker. We all dealt with Grandpa's cancer in our own personal way. My grandma was simply in denial, she simply and sincerely believed that grandpa would get better. My dad, my grandfather's only child took my grandfather's role and became the patriarch of our family. He wore a brave face.

Some of us felt betrayed by God and became hateful and hard.

Personally I began barraging with God. Every night I would pray,' Please God if you make grandpa better I will go to church every day. I will give my whole pay check away, or whatever you want." I thought I could bribe God into healing my grandpa.

My grandpa's illness was a very long and hard one. He was in and out of the hospital, in and out of hospice and finally put on life support. We watched this bigger than life man lose his independence, dignity and freedom. What I didn't realize is that God was giving him his freedom back!

As caregivers we learned that a point has to come that you have to let go of your loved one so they can have peace. You learn to accept God's will. You learn that becoming angry or bitter or tears just don't work.

My grandfather, in his last days taught us that the ultimate gift you can give someone is love. You can give them the gift of acceptance. Accept that no one lives forever, accept that cancer rob you of the love you have for that person, accept that dying is just another form of living and accept that your loved one will be ok, as long as you are ok!

When my grandfather was dying we used to look at family pictures whenever we were together. As we looked at those pictures I did not know until after he was gone that each time I remember him, I was celebrating his life. I am letting the light of HIS spirit shine in the world.

Chapter 3

As a caregiver I personally learned that peace only comes for your loved ones and yourself when you learn to accept what must be. When you waste your time being bitter or angry you are taking time, precious time away from your loved one.

"A caregiver's prayer"

Lord I pray your angels give me strength when I am weak. A friend to hold me when I am alone. A peaceful and accepting heart when you call my loved one home. Let my loved one's legacy shine in my eyes, let their kind gentle words live in my heart and through my actions. Amen.

"It is when God appears to abandon us that we must abandon ourselves solely to him." F. Fenelon

When my grandfather died it was like my grandma did also. My grandfather passed away on July 5, 1995. He was finally set free when my grandma signed a DNR order after weeks of praying for God to give our family wisdom and strength to do the right thing.

The day my grandfather passed, it was a brutally hot and miserable summer's day. Ironically or perhaps mercifully we got to the hospital to see my grandfather late that day. For weeks we had been going to the hospital at a set time to visit him

It was on that day, my mother a caregiver for the mentally ill had to work overtime at her job. We waited for mom to get out of work so we could all go to see grandpa together.

When we got to the fourth floor of the Hospital, the door to my grandfather's room was tightly shut.

A young nurse approached us with a grim face saying, I am sorry Fred passed away about an hour ago." Grandma fell apart. Having a heart condition we were afraid she would collapse. After calming her down we called the rest of our family to share the sad news.

One by one they came to the hospital. We all went into grandpa's room together. To our surprise Grandpa looked so at peace. The machines he was hooked up to for so long had been removed. He looked like he was sleeping. Slowly we said." Goodbye."

As we were planning my grandpa's wake, my mom, grandma and I got one more ultimate gift of love from not only God but grandpa. We had gone into a flower shop to pick out the flowers for the wake.

My grandma loved flowers. Her backyard looked like a botanical garden. My grandpa's favorite colors were yellow and red. After we picked out the flowers and paid for them we were walking out of the flower shop when the owner called us back in. He handed my grandma and mom yellow roses and me a red one. We had not told him that was my grandfather's favorite colors!

My grandma in her very deep pain did not see what we saw in the gift of those flowers until weeks later. My grandfather had a full military funeral on July 7, 1995 and was buried in Calverton National Cemetery on Long Island N.Y.

After we buried grandpa, grandma felt alone in a crowded room. She could not stop crying, everywhere she went memories of grandpa haunted her soul. Grandma became very depressed.

We were all worried about her. After a few months, grandma was not getting better. It was not until one day, when grandma was reading her bible that tears of mourning turned into healing rain. The scripture was John 14:1 ""Do not let your hearts be troubled. You believe in God; believe also in me."

Trust, we must trust in our tears. As caregivers our tears are not a sign of weakness or even mourning. Our tears can be a sign of acceptance, of healing and peace. It is acceptable to cry. It is a gift to let our loved ones cry. As caregivers it is very important to have an outlet for our fears. Seek out others to talk to if you are feeling overwhelmed, need advice or just need a shoulder to cry on. As much as we want to be superman we are not. We are only human.

We must also keep in mind, as caregivers that we must let our loved ones express their feelings. Even though it may be hard for us to hear. Let your loved ones talk about their fears, their wishes, and their levies. It is even healthy to have a good cry together.

Chapter 4

"Once you choose hope anything is possible." Christopher Reeve.

Hope! It is a cancer patient's secret weapon against gloomy and lonely days.

As my great uncle Willie laid in a hospital dying of lung cancer, hope became his best friend. Like my grandfather, my grandfather was a strong and proud man. He was a hard worker who provided for his family. Uncle Willie was a former butcher, at one time in his younger days he drove a team of horses. Uncle Willie was 85 years old when he was diagnosed with lung cancer. Like my grandfather he was quickly losing his fight.

As his body weakened his mind did not. Uncle Willie formulated a plan to provide for his family after he passed, to leave us hope after he was gone. As we visited with my dying uncle day he reminded us how special we were to him and God.

He shared with us family history he only knew. History to be passed down. As caregivers it is important to be bearers of our family roots, family history and stories. It is important to our loved ones to know our family history will live on.

As caregivers we can preserve our family history by making scrapbooks, recording our loved ones, writing our loved ones thoughts on paper, or making photo albums. It helps our loved ones to know that Hope will be passed down. My uncle had a very short battle with cancer, but the lesson we learned from his cancer is that everyone needs hope.

Our family histories contain stories of hope. Hope of seeing our dreams successes, hope of finding that special someone. Hope that our children will grow up happy and healthy.

"You have to live life. Not think about it. Step into the mist of things. Try and fail. Stand and love. Learn and Forgive. Be daring and never live in fear." This is the lesson I learned from my bubbly and faithful friend Diana while she was going through her battle with liver cancer.

Diana and I met while working together in a Collage café. Diana was this incredible loving soul who had a young heart, gave the best advice and made a to die for chicken salad. Diana was the head cook at the café. When Diana told me she had liver cancer I was at a loss for words. I didn't know what to say or how to act around Diana. I immediately feel into a caregiver role.

Diana was a very independent woman. She was a walker, who walked five miles a day, she was much older than me but I never knew it. When Diana got sick I started to mother and smother her. I began to crowd her. This independent woman started to resent how I was treating her. She did not want to be babied.

One day when I was visiting Diana at her apartment, I began to take care of her. I was picking up a pile of her dirty wash, Diana got mad at me saying," Why are you treating me like this?" Turning to Diana, I answered honestly," Because you are sick."

Loving Diana sat me down." Patti, sometimes the best thing you can do for a person with cancer is nothing at all. Sometimes being with them is all they need." She said.

At that moment Diana's words penetrated my thick skull. People with cancer still want their independence. They don't want their choices to be taken away just because they are sick. Sometimes as caregivers we tend to think we most do everything for those with cancer but that just isn't true.

People with cancer want to keep their freedom for as long as they can.

As caregivers we must respect their right to choose. Choose their own decisions about their health care, doctors, final wishes and other important things. Sometimes we need to just back off and give our loved ones space. Sometimes the best thing we can do is really nothing at all.

Diana's World Famous Chicken Salad

2. Pkgs. Of boneless chicken breasts.

1 large onion chopped.

4 stalks of finely chopped celery.

2 large tomatoes sliced.

4 teaspoons of honey.

3 teaspoons of Italian dressing.

1 dill pickle chopped fine.

6 tablespoons of mayonnaise.

Cook chicken in a pot of boiling water for an hour.

Let chicken cool for 30 min.

Dice chicken

In a large mixing bowl add all together.

Let chill one hour before serving.

Chapter 5

"He placed me in a little cage away from Garden's fair but I must sing the sweetest song because he placed me there. Not beat my wings against the cage if not my maker's will but raise my voice to Heaven's gate and sing the louder still." Kyle Sweet

This was the inspirational poem my dear friend Kyle recited over and over again to help her get through the pain of living with ovarian cancer. Kyle and I never met in person. She was the wife of Christian rock singer Michael Sweet of Stryper. A band I loved growing up.

Kyle was my pen pal. The big sister I never had. Our friendship bloomed from being pen pals to spiritual sisters.

Kyle Rae Sweet was a very spiritual, giving, kind, and loving person. When I was going through tough times in my life Kyle and her husband reached out to me and was truly an example of Christ's love on earth.

Although I was not a direct caregiver to Kyle, I learned many lessons from her battle with cancer. Unlike the other people I have known with cancer her battle was a very public one.

Kyle had to fight cancer every day with reporters and cameras, and fans surrounding her. Being a famous make-up artist who worked on such movies as Teen Wolf and the wife of Rock God Kyle could have wallowed in self-pity but she did not. Kyle, my dear friend used her battle to help others.

Kyle talked openly about her struggle. She shared all she was dealing with. Through the sale of her husband's cd," Touched" She raised money for cancer research and money for the Dana Faber Cancer Center.

Kyle became an inspiration to not only her friends but to people around the world.

Kyle used music. Poems and scripture to touch people and to heal the hearts of the broken hearted.

Kyle's spirit, her warmth, her generosity will live on for many years to come. Because I was not living in the same state as Kyle I was not able to be a direct caregiver for her physical needs but I was able to be a spiritual caregiver. How you ask?

We don't need to be with the person to be a caregiver, we can be a caregiver for their emotional, spiritual or even financial needs.

For Kyle I became a prayer giver. I prayed for Kyle at a certain time every single day. Sometimes the most powerful gift we can give someone is pray for them.

To listen, is a gift all in itself. If you have a friend or loved one going through this battle and you can't be with them physically there are still other ways to help.

Another way I supported Kyle was through writing encouraging cards and letters to her.

For someone battling cancer sometimes a simple gift of love, like receiving a card or letter is a way of hugging them even when you can't be there.

Below here are some other suggestions on how you can help.

1. Send the family a gift card to a local food store so they can eat and share a special meal together.
2. If the patient is going for treatments buy them a new bathrobe and some new slippers. This will make them feel like a million bucks.
3. A lot of people don't know that if a person is going for treatments they can't wear perfume or be around a lot of different smells, Flowers are nice, but sometimes it makes a person sick, so instead of buying flowers buy a cd player so they can play their favorite music.

4. If the person has a child send a gift card for a movie, then arrange for a babysitter to take the child to the movies so the patient and partner can have some quiet time together.

5. Offer to pay for a maid service so the caregiver will have one less thing to worry about.

6. If involved with a church organize some people to do yard work or cook some meals.

7. Offer to pay for a tank full of gas for the family to go to the doctors.

8. Pay for tolls or a parking garage for the day.

9. Offer to pay for one medical supply

10. **Offer to sit with the patient for an hour or two so the caregiver can get some rest.**

11. **Start a go-fund me page. Cancer not only takes your life but your money.**

These are little steps you can take to help a loved one far away.

The following list is where you can send a love gift to kick cancer's ass!

1. Dana Farber 10 Brookline Place West, 6TH floor Brookline M.A. 02445 ATTN. Partners in Courage.

2. Breast Cancer research. 60 East 56th Street. 8th Floor N.Y.N.Y. 10022

Side note: This is a revised version of this book. As I write this Kyle's mother-in-law Janice Sweet is now also batting cancer. Some of us Stryper fans have set up a go-fund I account to help her. If you wish to donate, the link is...

https://www.gofundme.com/nzr1nk

Anything will help this woman of God.

Chapter 6

Romans 15:13 new international version

"May the God of hope fill you with all joy and peace as you trust in him, so that you may overflow with hope by the power of the Holy Spirit?"

When I met my husband Anthony, we were working together at a factory. Just two weeks later, Anthony left the factory to work at another job. We lost contact. Ten years later we met again on a blind date.

We had our 1st date at Ruby Tuesdays. During our first date we discovered we had many things in common. We feel in love quickly and got engaged just two months later.

The first time I met Anthony's big, traditional Italian family, I feel in love with all of them. Anthony's family became a part of who I was. They became a part of my heart. Sometimes I think the best part of me.

Anthony and I wed on Oct 17, 1999 in a small country-style church on the East end of Long Island. It was the perfect fall day. The leaves had begun changing colors. There was a chill in the air. Fall embraced us like an old friend.

On that perfect day I walked down the aisle with both my parents in my long and flowing white gown as my church's choir director sang," Ava Maria." I saw the faces of my loved ones beaming with love, light and joy.

Two of those faces were my mom's older sister Roberta and my hubby's uncle Al. Both of them were loving souls, both of them had cancer.

Aunt Roberta had bone cancer. Uncle Al did as well. At my wedding both sides of the family were blessed to make so many happy memories that day. It was on that day that I found out that Anthony's sister was going to have a baby.

It was also at the wedding that both Aunt Roberta and Uncle Al were able to enjoy this wonderful, carefree and happy times with family and friends.

As caregivers it is so very important and crucial for us to realize that our loved ones need a very strong support system. A system that includes family, friends, church members, co-workers and classmates. We need to allow them to visit.

As caregivers we need to put our personal differences aside with other family members who the sake of those suffering cancer!

It is not about us, it is about them!

It is important for us to realize that if the patient wants to travel, go to a family event, visit a friend, go to class or church, they should not be limited to do so.

As caregivers we tend to protect and preserve our loved one's energy for fear if they overexert themselves or get upset they may get sicker or die. Not true!

If the patient wants to go have a picnic, go swimming in the Ocean, go to a party, or a concert let them! It is good for their soul. It is so important that they are not reminded 24/7 that they have cancer.

We must learn that we can't control cancer by controlling our loved ones! Our loved ones should not have to stop living because our fears prevent them from doing so!

Chapter 7

"The bond that links your true family is not of blood but of respect and joy in each other's life." Richard Bach.

Everyone has someone in their life that inspires them for greatness. For me personally, it is God, my Parents and my fourth grade teacher Mrs. Estevez.

Growing up I was a special education student. I had dyslexia. I was picked on, bullied and didn't have a lot of self-confidence. That was until Mrs. E came into my life.

Mrs. E saw in me a gift of writing. Mrs. E fueled my passion for writing by encouraging me and helping me overcome my disability.

She was a real friend. Someone who give the shirt off her back to help someone. She was a great teacher.

Long after I became a H.S. and Collage grad, Mrs. Estevez and her husband kept in touch with me. They even came to my wedding!

Once spring morning, I went to my mailbox and found a letter from Mrs. E Inside. Getting one of her letters always left me with a warm and fuzzy feeling. With the expectation of this letter. My heart sunk as I read the words," Mr. E has been diagnosed with blood cancer."

I ran into the house crying and shaking. Because yet another loved one had cancer. Damn Cancer!

I broke the tragic news to my husband and parents. We all had a good cry. Tossing and turning that night in my bed, I couldn't sleep. Something in Mrs. E's letter ate away at me. She didn't want me to write her anymore. I didn't understand why. What had I done wrong?

"Good friends are like stars. You don't always see them, but always know they are there." Unknown

For weeks I was depressed that Mrs. E was shutting me out at a time she needed her friends the most. I had written her and called her but never got a reply. Her silence tore apart my heart. I prayed for her and her husband. I wanted God to give me the answer. Why didn't she want me in her life anymore? The answer I was seeking came in a rare and unexpected way.

One of my old classmates had looked me up on Facebook. She had been a classmate that was once a very big part of my life. But we no longer had anything in common. As I listened to my classmate ramble on about her boring job, I realized Mrs. E was not trying to hurt me when she wrote that final letter. We were a beautiful part of each other's past but now we were facing two very different futures.

Mrs. E was becoming a full time caregiver trying to squeeze in every last moment she could with her husband. I was trying down a very different road. My future was full of dreams and plans.

Mrs. E's future was full of worry, sacrifice and taking care of a sick husband.

I learned from Mr. E's cancer that sometimes the most loving thing you can do is step out of a person's life and give them the space they need while they are going through this journey. Sometimes they just need time. Sometimes they just need to be alone. Sometimes they just need time to find their way through the haze of pain and maze of confusion.

I didn't hear from Mrs. Estevez for two solid years. And then one day, I opened my mailbox to find a letter from her.

Mr. E had gone to be with the Lord. Mrs. E had found her way back to the person she was before cancer put her life on hold. I know it's not easy to see someone struggling with the beast and to have them shut you out. It may seem like they are being selfish or mean, but they are not.

"Jesus healed many who had illness." Mark 1:34

Sometimes the most important lessons in life are the most painful. In the process of writing this book, I met a man, a stranger on the Street who touched my heart so deeply that I could not let this moment pass without mentioning him. His name is Peter. Peter was probably in his early 30s. He was in a wheelchair. He had lived through 7 different types of cancer.

From the moment I met Peter, I felt his positive vibe. Peter was a big brother, he ran his own company, and bought wheelchairs for people who couldn't afford them. In front of a Christian book store where I met Peter, he taught me a lesson in forgiveness.

As we chatted, Peter revealed to me that when he was diagnosed with cancer, his wife could not deal with it and left him for another man.

When I asked Peter if he was able to forgive his wife, he looked me dead in the eye and replied," If Jesus was able to forgive my sins, why shouldn't I forgive the sins of another?"

As we talked about forgiveness, Peter revealed to me how important it was to him to know he had forgiven all the people in his life that had hurt him and for them to forgive him to.

This brings me to a very important point, as caregivers, I think we need to make sure the people we are taking care of knows that we have forgiven them for past hurts, makes and grudges.

Forgiveness is very powerful. If you have a terminal illness, and feel like you have unforgivness in your heart towards someone or like you need to be forgiven, reach out. Don't let your heart be filled with turmoil. Otherwise you won't be at peace.

Chapter 8

Prayer of St. Frances." Lord, make me an instrument of thy peace. Where there is hatred, let me sow love; where there is injury, pardon; where there is doubt, faith;

Where there is despair, hope; where there is darkness, light; where there is sadness, joy.

O divine Master, grant that I may not so much seek To be consoled as to console, To be understood as to understand, To be loved as to love; For it is in giving that we receive; It is in pardoning that we are pardoned; It is in dying to self that we are born to eternal life."

"Humor is a way of defending ourselves from Life's absurdities by thinking absurdly about them." Lewis Mumford

"I am going to the hospital to deliver my twins." My co-worker and best friend Jane hood said as she spoke of having her breasts removed. Jane was diagnosed with cancer one January day right before coming to work at the Day Care where we both worked. Where we worked with two-year-olds.

Jane who always wore a smile on her face, had a song in her heart and a spring in her step casually broke the news to us with a positive attitude and laughter. Lots of laughter.

When Jane told us about her cancer, it was hard not to believe that she would not drag the beast by the hair, look it straight in the eye and tell it to go to Hell. Jane would overcome cancer and would use laughter to kick its butt!

Jane kept us all positive. She taught us it was ok to laugh at cancer. She taught us just because a person has cancer, it doesn't mean it has to be a death sentence. She taught us God is in control.

It was Jane that actual held her circle of friends together. She would not let us fall apart. After Jane lost her breasts, I went to see her and she had me laughing. Laughter really is the best medicine. I truly believe that it was the laughter of her friends and family that kept her strong even when she could have feel apart.

As I wrote the first version of this book, Jane had been cancer free for five years, but in 2016 on Mother's Day Jane passed away due to bone cancer. Her husband Larry, her children and 23 grandchildren and her legacy of laughter is what she left behind.

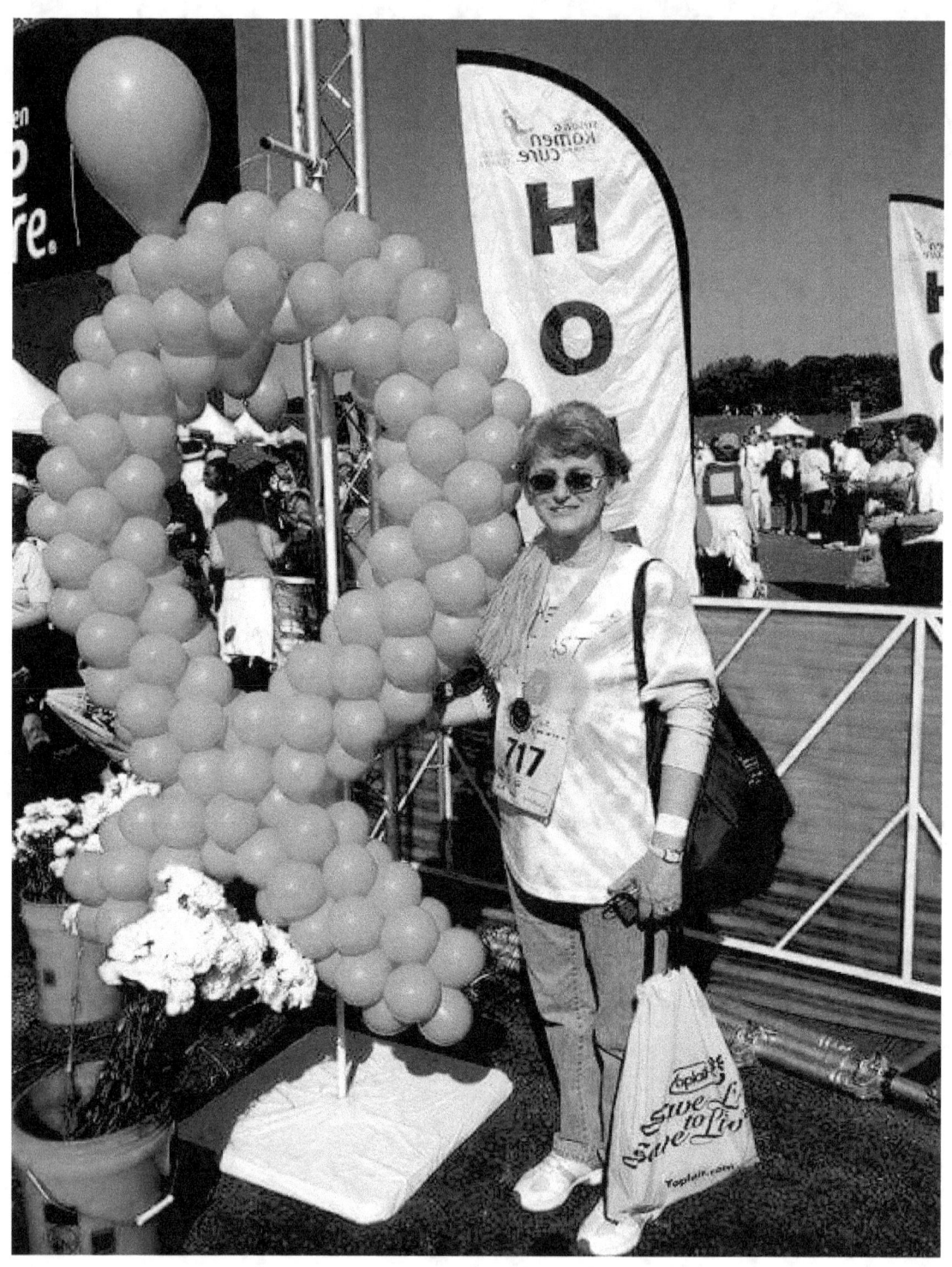

My dear friend Jane Hood- The one that made my soul Laugh.

Chapter 9

"God Heals Remember when you heard the words - and your mind went blank - you were in another world God heals Remember in your darkest hours - when all that surrounds you is pain and sorrow God heals Remember friends' prayers - your family's encouragement - glimmers of hope from every day angels God heals Quiet...you can hear Him now - always there - yet never this close God heals It's just another day - yet everything has changed - and you hear yourself say God heals Birds are singing - the sky is a beautiful blue - flowers are blooming...God heals Truths that you knew as a child - awakened again with new understanding

God heals Remember when others can't - that life is a gift - each day to treasure God Has Healed"

Breast Cancer resources.

City of Hope Cancer Center- Los Angeles, C.A. 1-800-826-4673

Memorial Sloan- N.Y 1-800-525-2225

Cancer support groups

4th Angel Mentoring Program

866-520-3197

http://www.4thangel.org

Air Charity Network

800-549-9980

http://www.aircharitynetwork.org

AMC Cancer Fund

303-233-6501

 800-321-1557

http://www.amc.org/

American Association for Cancer Research (AACR)

215-440-9300

Toll Free: 866-423-3965

http://www.aacr.org

American Cancer Society

404-320-3333

Toll Free: 800-ACS-2345

TTY: 866-288-4327

http://www.cancer.org

American Cancer Society Cancer Action Network (ACS CAN)

800-ACS-2345

http://www.acscan.org

American Hospice Foundation

202-223-0204

800-347-1413

http://www.americanhospice.org

American Society for Radiation Oncology703-502-1550

 1-800-962-7876

http://www.astro.org/Patient

American Society of Breast Surgeons

410-992-5470

 1-877-992-5470

http://www.breastsurgeons.org

Anderson Network, a Program of Volunteer Services

800-345-6324

http://www.mdanderson.org/andersonnetwork

Arab Community Center for Economic and Social Services (ACCESS)

313-842-7010

http://www.accesscommunity.org

Association of Cancer Online Resources

http://www.acor.orgAssociation of Community Cancer Centers (ACCC)

301-984-9496

http://www.accc-cancer.org

Cancer Family Relief Fund

415-887-8932

http://www.cancerfamilyrelieffund.org

Cancer Financial Assistance Coalition

http://www.cancerfac.org

Chapter 10

"When you were born you cried and the world rejoiced. Live your life to the fullest so when you die, the world cries and you rejoice." Old Indian expression.

Dad, Father, Pop, Daddy are all words that make you feel secure, warmed, loved and happy. My father, my friend, hero, my teacher, my confident advisor, Bernie Leudeman was a man who had no regrets. He loved, He lived, and He gave with all his heart.

When I think of my father, The Frank Sinatra song, My Way comes to mind. My father was passionate about life. He was a hard worker, faithful friend, loving father and devoted husband. He loved gardening just like his mom. He loved animals just like St. Frances. He loved fast cars, fish and music.

Dad wore many hats. He started his working career selling pretzels at Madison Square Garden. Became a proud business owner and finally retired from Pilgrim State Hospital on Long Island in the late 1990s.

Dad and Mom met on a blind date. They got married on Aug, 22, 1970.

Dad was nick named," The Bull." Because he was a strong man with a gentle heart. He had a booming voice, blue eyes and blond hair. He was born on Oct 25, 1942 in Brooklyn, N.Y. and died Sept 27,

2006 in Covington G.A. He was another victim of the damn beast.

My dad's death was untimely, shocking, and the most painful for my family. After my parents retired from their jobs in N.Y. they headed down south. Dad always loved cowboys and westerns so moving to the Deep South was a dream come true for him.

"It matters not who you love, where you love, why you love, or how you love. All that matters is that you love." John Lennon.

My parents purchased a charming 3 bedroom 2 bath ranch with a huge backyard in the lovely little town of Covington. The town where the Dukes of Hazard was filmed. My parents quickly became adopted southern. Dad loved working in his flower garden, playing with his dogs and sitting on his porch listening to Country songs. Dad was the picture of perfect health.

In the summer of 2006 my husband and I planned a family reunion. It was my parent's 36 wedding anniversary coming up and my niece's birthday.

My in-laws, brother and a friends flew up from New York for the big family reunion. The family spent the week together, touring all the sites, going out and just having a wonderful time together. Dad was fine.

On the day of my parent's anniversary we had a fun celebration. We ate fine food, drank, listened to music and danced. It was a happy time for all of us.

When the week came to an end we were sad to see the rest of our family go but we knew we would see them soon enough for the Christmas Holiday. On the way home from dropping our guests off at the airport, my dad who was driving started to complain of shoulder pain.

He thought it was arthritis. Dad went home and rested.

The next day my husband and I went to work. When we got home there was a message from mom saying," I think your father had a stroke, He can't move his arm or leg." My husband and I jumped in the car and drove to my parents' home.

We tried to get dad to go to the Hospital but he just brushed it off.

Later that night dad got worse. He couldn't walk and was having really bad headaches. We called 911. At the hospital, the doctors ran all kinds of tests on dad. I will never forget the moment the doctor came into the room and told us my dad had brain cancer. Everything stopped. I recall hearing screams and I didn't realize those screams were coming from my own mouth. My husband passed out. My mom turned white as a ghost. Then I recall dad. The rock of our family.

"How long do I have?" Dad asked the doctor.

The young doctor looked at me and my husband, who had his arms wrapped tightly around me. "Maybe a week." The young doctor said." I want to go home and die." Dad said to Mom.

Later on that night, my brother flew down to G.A. I recall how destroyed he was. We sat in silence as we drove back to my parents' house together to wait for Hospice to set up a hospital bed for dad. My brother and I couldn't look at each other. There were no words to say that could have comforted us.

Hospice came. I feel apart. Mom, my brother and husband remained strong. My dad made it clear to us, his final wishes. He told us everything he needed to say. There were no words left unspoken between us. No tears unshed. We had our pastor give dad last rites.

One week to the day, dad died. We were unprepared for his death, financially and emotionally.

When dad died, we had both a Catholic Priest and Methodist one send dad's soul back to God.

Dad was buried in N.Y. next to his parents. After dad died, I felt lost, betrayed and very lonely. I was not mentally prepared to lose my dad. I had a really hard time getting over his death.

Talking about my dad helped. Going to places we used to go together helped. Having a picture of my dad on the dashboard of my car helped.

The most important lesson, I learned from my dad's death is that you are never alone in your grief. There are always people out there that can help.

Everyone goes through the grieving process differently. No one has the right to tell you to stop mourning. I don't care if has been one day or ten years since you have lost your loved one, there is no set amount of time that is normal or not normal to grieve.

The same things goes for if you have been diagnosed with cancer. Another lesson I learn was no matter how much pain you are in, life will go on.

There are seven stages of grief. They are as follows.

SHOCK & DENIAL-

You will probably react to learning of the loss with numbed disbelief. You may deny the reality of the loss at some level, in order to avoid the pain. Shock provides emotional protection from being overwhelmed all at once. This may last for weeks.

2. PAIN & GUILT-

As the shock wears off, it is replaced with the suffering of unbelievable pain. Although excruciating and almost unbearable, it is important that you experience the pain fully, and not hide it, avoid it or escape from it with alcohol or drugs.

You may have guilty feelings or remorse over things you did or didn't do with your loved one. Life feels chaotic and scary during this phase.

3. ANGER & BARGAINING-

Frustration gives way to anger, and you may lash out and lay unwarranted blame for the death on someone else. Please try to control this, as permanent damage to your relationships may result. This is a time for the release of bottled up emotion.

You may rail against fate, questioning "Why me?" You may also try to bargain in vain with the powers that be for a way out of your despair ("I will never drink again if you just bring him back")

4."DEPRESSION", REFLECTION, LONELINESS-

Just when your friends may think you should be getting on with your life, a long period of sad reflection will likely overtake you. This is a normal stage of grief, so do not be "talked out of it" by well-meaning outsiders. Encouragement from others is not helpful to you during this stage of grieving.

During this time, you finally realize the true magnitude of your loss, and it depresses you. You may isolate yourself on purpose, reflect on things you did with your lost one, and focus on memories of the past. You may sense feelings of emptiness or despair.

More 7 stages of grief...

5. THE UPWARD TURN-

As you start to adjust to life without your dear one, your life becomes a little calmer and more organized. Your physical symptoms lessen, and your "depression" begins to lift slightly.

6. RECONSTRUCTION & WORKING THROUGH-

As you become more functional, your mind starts working again, and you will find yourself seeking realistic solutions to problems posed by life without your loved one. You will start to work on practical and financial problems and reconstructing yourself and your life without him or her.

7. ACCEPTANCE & HOPE-

During this, the last of the seven stages in this grief model, you learn to accept and deal with the reality

of your situation. Acceptance does not necessarily mean instant happiness. Given the pain and turmoil you have experienced, you can never return to the carefree, untroubled YOU that existed before this tragedy. But you will find a way forward.

You will start to look forward and actually plan things for the future. Eventually, you will be able to think about your lost loved one without pain; sadness, yes, but the wrenching pain will be gone. You will once again anticipate some good times to come, and yes, even find joy again in the experience of living.

What can you do if you have lost a loved one or have been diagnosed with cancer?

Here are several suggestions to help you.

1. Get sleep.
2. Exercise if you can
3. Make sure you eat
4. Avoid drugs and alcohol
5. Join a support group.

It is very important in this difficult time that you get sleep. If you wake up feeling tried your mind won't be capable of helping you heal. You will find yourself more irritable, more depressed and more sensitive. Sleep helps you to relax and heal your mind.

Exercise if you can. Exercise could be the key to healing. It releases tension and stress. It will help you forget your pain.

Eat right. I know it can be difficult for you to eat right now but your body needs food. Grief expends an enormous amount of energy. Without food you will get run down and weak.

Avoid drugs and drink. It may help you forget your pain for a while, but the truth is it won't bring your loved one back or make your cancer go away.

Join a support group. There is no shame in admitting you are in pain.

The following are some examples of how to honor a loved one that has died.

1. Plant a flower garden in your loved ones memory. For every birthday plant a new flower in the garden.

2. Collect funny stories, pictures, and memories from family, friends, co-workers, classmates and make a scrapbook honoring all the love you have for that person.

3. Set aside a special place and time to talk to your loved one every day. They are not just a memory. Your loved one lives on in your soul!

4. Donate to their favorite charity.

5. Don't stop celebrating your loved ones birthday, anniversary or any special day. They lived and loved and you should celebrate that!

As my family and loved ones were going through this joinery we found that music really helped us on the days we were discouraged. The following is a list of songs, my loved ones used to listen too as they were going through treatment, songs we used to give us peace and to summon our guardian angels.

1. A wonderful World by Louis Armstrong

2. Somewhere over the rainbow by Judy Garland
3. It's a beautiful day by U2
4. It's my life by Bon Jovi.
5. Ture Colors By Cyndi Lauper
6. She's got a way By Billy Joel
7. Honestly By Stryper
8. Friends by Michael. W. Smith.
9. 9. Peace in the Valley by Elvis
10. I'm too sexy by Right said Fred.

Chapter 11

"Courage doesn't always roar. Sometimes courage is the quiet voice at the end of the day saying, "I will try again tomorrow." Mary Anne Radmacher

As I mentioned before, this is a revised version of this book. I have to share my own story with a cancer scare.

In late 2013 I was a hardworking 40 year old with two full time jobs. I was a teacher for two fabulous day cares. I was happy, healthy and full of life. But in one tragic turn of events my life changed drastically. I had a stroke. ALL-through I was in I.C.U. for 5 days I considered myself blessed because I was still able to speak, hear, see and comprehend. With time and pt. I recovered from my stroke, but then another health crisis. At the end of 2013 my doctor found a tumor growing inside my fema bone. I was sent to an orthopedic oncologist and he said I needed surgery and a biopsy right away. I trusted the doctor and placed his life in my hands. My family and I were very scared because we had lost 14 people to cancer. After a 6 hour surgery, 5 blood transfusions and years of pain, my leg has not been the same. There is a back story here. You see the doctor that had done my leg surgery was sued for malpractice not by me but by seven other people who lost their limbs. The doctor who actually did my leg surgery has skipped the country. My surgery was a Failure. I now have permeant nerve damage in my leg and I have to use a scooter everywhere I go, because my leg can't hold my body weight nor can I walk around with the 8 inch hole that I have in my fema bone. No doctor and I have been to many will touch my leg now. But my story doesn't end there. In 2014 I had a second stroke this time it was worse. I have a bit of memory issues and my right hand was left weak. We found out last year in 2015 that the strokes were caused by undiagnosed Lupus. I am now on meds to control my pain, the lupus and five recently diagnosed blood clots I have in my leg. I am NOT writing this to have anyone feel sorry for me. I am alive. But I am writing this as a warning. I do not know to this day, if I had/ have cancer in my leg. You see the doctor when he skipped the country, skipped with all my medical files, my biopsy, pictures and MRI's of my leg and everything else that goes along with it.

I am living through Hell. Every six weeks, I have to get an MRI on my leg, ordered by my new orthopedic oncologist, yes I am being treated by a CANCER doctor to see if there have been any" changes" to my fema bone. I am also on heavy pain medication because I have an eight inch hole in my bone and the rod the doctor put in (the doctor that took off on me) is through major nerves in my leg.

Another example I must share with you of doctor's failing is, my cousin Diane was diagnosed with ovarian cancer, after months and months of doctors not doing anything she passed away. By the time they found the cancer it was stage four and she passed on.

So why is this nightmarish chapter being added to the book? It is a warning, KNOW WHO YOUR DOCTOR IS!

Research them. If you can't personally research them, ask a family or friend to do it.

When choosing a doctor for your cancer care, you may find it helpful to know some of the terms used to describe a doctor's training and credentials. Most physicians who treat people with cancer are medical doctors (they have an M.D. degree) or osteopathic doctors (they have a D.O. degree). The basic training for both types of physicians includes 4 years of premedical education at a college or university, 4 years of medical school to earn an M.D. or D.O. degree, and postgraduate medical education through internships and residences. This training usually lasts 3 to 7 years. Physicians must pass an exam to become licensed (legally permitted) to practice medicine in their state. Each state or territory has its own procedures and general standards for licensing physicians.

Specialists are physicians who have completed their residency training in a specific area, such as internal medicine. Independent specialty boards certify physicians after they have fulfilled certain requirements. These requirements include meeting specific education and training criteria, being licensed to practice medicine, and passing an examination given by the specialty board. Doctors who have met all of the requirements are given the status of "Diplomate" and are board certified as specialists. Doctors who are bored eligible have obtained the required education and training but have not completed the specialty board examination.

After being trained and certified as a specialist, a physician may choose to become a subspecialist. A subspecialist has at least 1 additional year of full-time education in a particular area of a specialty. This training is designed to increase the physician's expertise in a specific field. Specialists can be board certified in their subspecialty as well.

The following are some specialties and subspecialties that pertain to cancer treatment:

• **Medical Oncology is a subspecialty of internal medicine.** Doctors who specialize in internal medicine treat a wide range of medical problems. Medical oncologists treat cancer and manage the patient's course of treatment. A medical oncologist may also consult with other physicians about the patient's care or refer the patient to other specialists.

• **Hematology is a subspecialty of internal medicine.** Hematologists focus on diseases of the blood and related tissues, including the bone marrow, spleen, and lymph nodes.

• Radiation Oncology is a subspecialty of radiology. Radiology is the use of x-rays and other forms of radiation to diagnose and treat disease. Radiation oncologists specialize in the use of radiation to treat cancer.

• Surgery is a specialty that pertains to the treatment of disease by surgical operation. General surgeons perform operations on almost any area of the body. Physicians can also choose to specialize in a certain type of surgery; for example, thoracic surgeons are specialists who perform operations specifically in the chest area, including the lungs and the esophagus.

The American Board of Medical Specialties® (ABMS) is a not-for-profit organization that assists medical specialty boards with the development and use of standards for evaluation and certification of physicians. Information about other specialties that treat cancer is available from the ABMS website.

Almost all board-certified specialists are members of their medical specialty society. Physicians can attain Fellowship status in a specialty society, such as the American College of

Surgeons (ACS), if they demonstrate outstanding achievement in their profession. Criteria for Fellowship status may include the number of years of membership in the specialty society, years practicing in the specialty, and professional recognition by peers.

How can I find a doctor who specializes in cancer care?

One way to find a doctor who specializes in cancer care is to ask for a referral from your primary care physician. You may know a specialist yourself, or through the experience of a family member, coworker, or friend.

The following resources may also be able to provide you with names of doctors who specialize in treating specific diseases or conditions. However, these resources may not have information about the quality of care that the doctors provide.

• Your local hospital or its patient referral service may be able to provide you with a list of specialists who practice at that hospital.

• Your nearest NCI-designated cancer center can provide information about doctors who practice at that center. The NCI-Designated Cancer Centers Find a Cancer Center page provides contact information to help health care providers and cancer patients with referrals to NCI-designated cancer centers located throughout the United States.

• The ABMS has a list of doctors who have met certain education and training requirements and have passed specialty examinations. Is Your Doctor Board Certified Exit Disclaimer lists doctors' names along with their specialty and their educational background? Users must register to use this online self-serve resource, which allows users to conduct searches by a physician's name or area of certification and a state name. The directory is available in most libraries.

• The American Medical Association (AMA) Doctor Finder database provides basic information on licensed physicians in the United States. Users can search for physicians by name or by medical specialty.

• The American Society of Clinical Oncology (ASCO) provides an online list of doctors who are members of ASCO. The member database Exit Disclaimer has the names and affiliations of nearly 30,000 oncologists worldwide. It can be searched by doctor's name, institution, location, oncology specialty, and/or type of board certification.

• **The American College of Surgeons (ACS) membership database Exit Disclaimer** is an online list of surgeons who are members of the ACS. The list can be searched by doctor's name, geographic location, or medical specialty. The ACS can be contacted by telephone at 1-800-621-4111.

• **The American Osteopathic Association (AOA) Find a Doctor** database provides an online list of practicing osteopathic physicians who are AOA members. The information can be searched by doctor's name, geographic location, or medical specialty. The

AOA can be contacted by telephone at 1-800-621-1773.

• Local medical societies may maintain lists of doctors in each specialty.

• Public and medical libraries may have print directories of doctors' names listed geographically by specialty.

• Your local Yellow Pages or Yellow Book may have doctors listed by specialty under "Physicians."

If you are a member of a health insurance plan, your choice may be limited to doctors who participate in your plan. Your insurance company can provide you with a list of participating primary care doctors and specialists. It is important to ask whether the doctor you are considering is accepting new patients through your health plan. You also have the option of seeing a doctor outside your health plan and paying the costs yourself. If you have the option to change health insurance plans, you may first wish to consider which doctor or doctors you would like to use, and then choose a plan that includes your chosen physician(s).

If you are using a federal or state health insurance program such as Medicare or Medicaid, you may want to ask whether the doctor you are considering is accepting patients who use these programs.

You will have many factors to consider when choosing a doctor. To make an informed decision, you may wish to speak with several doctors before choosing one. When you meet with each doctor, you might want to consider the following:

• Does the doctor have the education and training to meet my needs?

• Does the doctor use the hospital that I have chosen?

• Does the doctor listen to me and treat me with respect?

• **Does the doctor explain things clearly and encourage me to ask questions?**

• **What are the doctor's office hours?**

• **Who covers for the doctor when he or she is unavailable? Will that person have access to my medical records?**

• **How long does it take to get an appointment with the doctor?**

If you are choosing a surgeon, you may wish to ask additional questions about the surgeon's background and experience with specific procedures. These questions may include:

- **Is the surgeon board certified?**

- **Has the surgeon been evaluated by a national professional association of surgeons, such as the ACS?**

- **At which treatment facility or facilities does the surgeon practice?**

- **How often does the surgeon perform the type of surgery I need?**

- **How many of these procedures has the surgeon performed? What was the success rate? It is important for you to feel comfortable with the specialist that you choose because you will be working closely with that person to make decisions about your cancer treatment. Trust your** own observations and feelings when deciding on a doctor for your medical care.

How can I get another doctor's opinion about the diagnosis and treatment plan?

After your doctor gives you advice about the diagnosis and treatment plan, you may want to get another doctor's opinion before you begin treatment. This is known as getting a second opinion. You can do this by asking another specialist to review all of the materials related to your case. The doctor who gives the second opinion can confirm or suggest modifications to your doctor's proposed treatment plan, provide reassurance that you have explored all of your options, and answer any questions you may have.

Getting a second opinion is done frequently, and most physicians welcome another doctor's views. In fact, your doctor may be able to recommend a specialist for this consultation. However, some people find it uncomfortable to request a second opinion. When discussing this issue with your doctor, it may be helpful to express satisfaction with your doctor's decision and care and to mention that you want your decision about treatment to be as thoroughly informed as possible. You may also wish to bring a family member along for support when asking for a second opinion. It is best to involve your doctor in the process of getting a second opinion, because your doctor will need to make your medical records (such as your test results and x-rays) available to the specialist who is giving the second opinion.

Some health care plans require a second opinion, particularly if a doctor recommends surgery. Other health care plans will pay for a second opinion if the patient requests it. If your plan does not cover a second opinion, you can still obtain one if you are willing to cover the cost.

If your doctor is unable to recommend a specialist for a second opinion, or if you prefer to choose one on your own, the following resources can help:

• Many of the resources listed above for finding a doctor can also help you find a specialist for a consultation.

• The NIH Clinical Center in Bethesda, Maryland, is the research hospital for the NIH, including NCI. Several branches of the NCI provide second opinion services. The NCI fact sheet Cancer Clinical Trials at the NIH Clinical Center describes these NCI branches and their services.

• The R. A. Bloch Cancer Foundation, Inc., can refer cancer patients to institutions that are willing to provide multidisciplinary second opinions. A list of these institutions is available on the organization's website. You can also contact the R. A. Bloch Cancer Foundation, Inc., by telephone at 816–854–5050 or 1–800–433–0464.

How can U.S. residents find treatment facilities?

Choosing a treatment facility is another important consideration for getting the best medical care possible. Although you may not be able to choose which hospital treats you in an emergency, you can choose a facility for scheduled and ongoing care. If you have already found a doctor for your cancer treatment, you may need to choose a facility based on where your doctor practices. Your doctor may be able to recommend a facility that provides quality care to meet your needs. You may wish to ask the following questions when considering a treatment facility:

• Has the facility had experience and success in treating my condition?

• Has the facility been rated by state, consumer, or other groups for its quality of care?

- **How does the facility check on and work to improve its quality of care?**

- **Has the facility been approved by a nationally recognized accrediting body, such as the ACS Commission on Cancer and/or The Joint Commission?**

- **Does the facility explain patients' rights and responsibilities? Are copies of this information available to patients?**

- **Does the treatment facility offer support services, such as social workers and resources, to help me find financial assistance if I need it?**

- **Is the facility conveniently located?**

If you are a member of a health insurance plan, your choice of treatment facilities may be limited to those that participate in your plan. Your insurance company can provide you with a list of approved facilities. Although the costs of cancer treatment can be very high, you do have the option of paying out-of-pocket if you want to use a treatment facility that is not covered by your insurance plan. If you are considering paying for treatment yourself, you may wish to discuss the possible costs with your doctor beforehand. You may also want to speak with the person who does the billing for the treatment facility. Nurses and social workers may also be able to provide you with more information about coverage, eligibility, and insurance issues.

The following resources may help you find a hospital or treatment facility for your care:

• The NCI-Designated Cancer Centers Find a Cancer Center page provides contact information for NCI-designated cancer centers located throughout the country.

• The ACS's Commission on Cancer (CoC) accredits cancer programs at hospitals and other treatment facilities. More than 1,430 programs in the United States have been designated by the CoC as

Approved Cancer Programs. The ACS website offers a searchable database Exit Disclaimer of these programs. The CoC can be contacted by telephone at 312–202–5085 or by e-mail at CoC@facs.org.

• The Joint Commission Exit Disclaimer is an independent not-for-profit organization that evaluates and accredits health care organizations and programs in the United States. It also offers information for the general public about choosing a treatment facility. The Joint Commission can be contacted by telephone at 630–792–5000.

The Joint Commission offers an online Quality Check Exit Disclaimer service that patients can use to determine whether a specific facility has been accredited by the Joint Commission and to view the organization's performance reports.

How can people who live outside the United States find treatment facilities in or near their countries?

If you live outside the United States, facilities that offer cancer treatment may be located in or near your country. Cancer information services are available in many countries to provide information and answer questions about cancer; they may also be able to help you find a cancer treatment facility close to where you live. A list of these cancer information services is available on the website of the International Cancer Information Service Group Exit Disclaimer, an independent international organization of cancer information services. A list may also be requested by writing to the NCI Public Inquiries Office at:

Cancer Information Service

BG 9609 MSC 9760

9609 Medical Center Drive

Bethesda, MD 20892-9760

USA

The Union for International Cancer Control (UICC) is another resource for people living outside the United States who want to find a cancer treatment facility. The UICC consists of international cancer-related organizations devoted to the worldwide fight against cancer. UICC membership includes research facilities and treatment centers and, in some countries, ministries of health. Other members include volunteer cancer leagues, associations, and societies. These organizations serve as resources for the public and may have helpful information about cancer and treatment facilities. To find a resource in or near your country, contact the UICC at:

Union for International Cancer Control (UICC)

62 route de Frontenex

1207 Geneva

Switzerland

+ 41 22 809 1811

http://www.uicc. How can people who live outside the United States get a second opinion or have cancer treatment in the United States?

Some people living outside the United States may wish to obtain a second opinion or have their cancer treatment in this country. Many facilities in the United States offer these services to international cancer patients. These facilities may also provide support services, such as language interpretation, assistance with travel, and guidance in finding accommodations near the treatment facility for patients and their families.

If you live outside the United States and would like to obtain cancer treatment in this country, you should contact cancer treatment facilities directly to find out whether they have an international patient office. The NCI-Designated Cancer Centers Find a Cancer Center page offers contact information for NCI-designated cancer centers throughout the United States.

Citizens of other countries who are planning to travel to the United States for cancer treatment generally must first obtain a nonimmigrant visa for medical treatment from the U.S. Embassy or Consulate in their home country. Visa applicants must demonstrate that the purpose of their trip is to enter the United States for medical treatment; that they plan to remain for a specific, limited period; that they have funds to cover expenses in the United States; that they have a residence and social and economic ties outside the United States; and that they intend to return to their home country.

To determine the specific fees and documentation required for the nonimmigrant visa and to learn more about the application process, contact the U.S. Embassy or Consulate in your home country. A list of links to the websites of U.S. Embassies and Consulates worldwide can be found on the U.S. Department of State's website.

Chapter 12

"Eating is so intimate. It's very sensual. When you invite someone to sit at your table and you want to cook for them, you're inviting a person into your life." Maya Angelou

Cancer diets can be very confusing. I know. Chemo and radiation wreak have on a body. You may feel very depressed and not want to eat. Here are a few suggestions on what to eat when you are going through treatments.

Fortified milk

Drink or use in place of milk in any recipe to add protein

1 quart whole or low-fat milk

1 cup powdered non-fat dry milk

Blend and chill at least 6 hours (can also be made with buttermilk or dry buttermilk).

Approximate nutrients per 1 cup serving: 211 calories and 14 grams of protein

Banana berry shake

4 scoops vanilla frozen yogurt

10 fresh strawberries

½ banana

Rinse strawberries. Put all ingredients in a blender and blend until smooth. Makes 2 servings.

Approximate nutrients per serving: 198 calories, 7 grams protein, 2 grams fat

Chocolate cocoa drink

1¼ cup vanilla ice cream

½ cup whole milk

1 package of hot chocolate mix

2 teaspoons sugar

Place all ingredients in a blender container. Cover and blend on high speed until well mixed.

Chill drinks before serving. Makes 2 servings.

Approximate nutrients per serving: 600 calories and 24 grams of protein per serving

Taco dip

1 16-ounce container sour cream

1 envelope taco seasoning

1 head lettuce, shredded

2 tomatoes, chopped

1 cup shredded cheddar cheese

1 package tortilla chips

Combine sour cream and taco seasoning in a small bowl and chill for 1 hour.

Take a large shallow dish and layer the ingredients, one by one, in the dish in the following order: sour cream mix, lettuce, tomatoes, and cheese.

Serve with tortilla chips for dipping. Makes 8 servings.

Approximate nutrients per serving: 483 calories, 10 grams protein, 31 grams fat

Peanut butter, banana, and raisin sandwich

2 tablespoons peanut butter

1 small banana, sliced

4 slices raisin bread

Spread peanut butter on 2 slices of bread. Arrange banana slices on top and cover with remaining bread.

Cut into quarters and serve. Makes 2 servings.

Approximate nutrients per serving: 278 calories, 9 grams protein, 11 grams fat

Peanut butter and jelly rounds

4 teaspoons creamy peanut butter

2 teaspoons grape jelly

8 Ritz® crackers

In a small bowl mix some peanut butter and jelly together until smooth.

Spread onto a Ritz cracker and top with another cracker to make sandwiches. Makes 2 servings.

Approximate nutrients per serving: 140 calories, 4 grams protein, 9 grams fat

Chapter 13

"Before you can live a part of you has to die. You have to let go of what could have been, how you should have acted and what you wish you would have said differently. You have to accept that you can't change the past experiences, opinions of others at that moment in time or outcomes from their choices or yours. When you finally recognize that truth then you will understand the true meaning of forgiveness of yourself and others. From this point you will finally be free."

— Shannon L. Alder

Cancer, it's an ugly word. Everything about Cancer is ugly.

There are many different types of cancer. There are over 2000 types. But do you know any of the signs of cancer?

Below are a list of signs to watch out for. Good to your doctor. Don't wait, the life you save could be your own!

Fatigue

• Lump or area of thickening that can be felt under the skin

• Weight changes, including unintended loss or gain

• Skin changes, such as yellowing, darkening or redness of the skin, sores that won't heal, or changes to existing moles

- Changes in bowel or bladder habits
- Persistent cough or trouble breathing
- Difficulty swallowing
- Hoarseness
- Persistent indigestion or discomfort after eating
- Persistent, unexplained muscle or joint pain
- Persistent, unexplained fevers or night sweats
- Unexplained bleeding or bruising

Chapter 14

"Prayer is not asking. It is a longing of the soul. It is daily admission of one's weakness. It is better in prayer to have a heart without words than words without a heart."

— Mahatma Gandhi

So you have cancer. Your loved one has been diagnosed. Do you pray they are cured? Do you pray for a peaceful death? Here are some scriptures and prayers that will help you through this must difficult time in your life.

Deuteronomy 31:6 "...Be strong and courageous. Do not fear or be in dread of them, for it is the Lord your God who goes with you. He will not leave you or forsake you."

Psalms 138:3 on the day I called, you answered me; my strength of soul you increased.

Proverbs 3:5-6 Trust in the LORD with all your heart, and do not lean on your own understanding. In all your ways acknowledge him, and he will make straight your paths.

Matthew 11:28-29 Come to me, all who labor and are heavy laden, and I will give you rest. Take my yoke upon you, and learn from me, for I am gentle and lowly in heart, and you will find rest for your souls.

2 Corinthians 1:3-4 Blessed be the God and Father of our Lord Jesus Christ, the Father of mercies and God of all comfort, who comforts us in all our affliction, so that we may be able to comfort those who are in any affliction, with the comfort with which we ourselves are comforted by God.

God is Faithful; calm for the Anxious

Psalms 18:6 in my distress I called upon the Lord; to my God I cried for help. From his temple he heard my voice, and my cry to him reached his ears.

Psalms 33:20-22 our soul waits for the LORD; he is our help and our shield. For our heart is glad in him, because we trust in his holy name. Let your steadfast love, O LORD, be upon us, even as we hope in you.

Philippians 1:6 And I am sure of this, that he who began a good work in you will bring it to completion at the day of Jesus Christ.

Philippians 4:6-7 ...do not be anxious about anything, but in everything by prayer and supplication with thanksgiving let your requests be made known to God. And the peace of God, which surpasses all understanding, will guard your hearts and your minds in Christ Jesus.

1 Peter 5:6-7 humble yourselves, therefore, under the mighty hand of God so that at the proper time he may exalt you, casting all your anxieties on him, because he cares for you.

God is Trustworthy; He Has a Plan for You

Ecclesiastes 3:1 for everything there is a season, and a time for every matter under heaven

Jeremiah 29:11 for I know the plans I have for you, declares the LORD, plans for welfare and not for evil, to give you a future and a hope.

John 14:1-3 "Let not your hearts be troubled. Believe in God; believe also in me. In my Father's house are many rooms. If it were not so, would I have told you that I go to prepare a place for you? And if I go and prepare a place for you, I will come again and will take you to myself, that where I am you may be also…"

God is Hope; Even When it Seems Hopeless

Romans 8:16-17 The Spirit himself bears witness with our spirit that we are children of God, and if children, then heirs—heirs of God and fellow heirs with Christ, provided we suffer with him in order that we may also be glorified with him.

Romans 8:24-25 for in this hope we were saved. Now hope that is seen is not hope. For who hopes for what he sees? But if we hope for what we do not see, we wait for it with patience.

Romans 8:38-39 For I am sure that neither death nor life, nor angels nor rulers, nor things present nor things to come, nor powers, nor height nor depth, nor anything else in all creation, will be able to separate us from the love of God in Christ Jesus our Lord.

1 Peter 1:3 blessed be the God and Father of our Lord Jesus Christ! According to his great mercy, he

has caused us to be born again to a living hope through the resurrection of Jesus Christ from the dead.

Dear Father.

Be with all those whose lives have been touched by cancer and who need strength to face each new day with hope and courage. Their hope is for recovery and many times this is granted but sometimes this is not to be and they have to accept whatever the future brings. Please hold them all in your hands, Lord, ease their fear and bring them your healing and wholeness.

Chapter 15

"We strive to find love and happiness. Life can be tough at times. I know that life can knock you into the dirt. I try to live each day as if I was going to die at the end of it."- Unknown

My daily diary

1.I am beautiful because......

2. I can beat cancer because.......

3. My battle with cancer will help others because......

4. Scriptures that encourage me are..........

5.My cancer battle song is...........

6.The reasons I will not give up are........

6. I have hope because.......

7. My prayer is.........

8. Lessons I learned from Cancer are....

9. A message I want to tell my family...........

10. Things that give me peace....

11. What I want the world to know about me.....

12. My final wishes....